Pocket Guide to OSCE

for the MRCOG

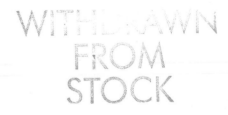

Pocket Guide to OSCE

for the MRCOG

Khaled M Khaled, Roopa Nair
and Barry Whitlow

RCOG PRESS 2006

Published by the RCOG Press at the
Royal College of Obstetricians and Gynaecologists
27 Sussex Place, Regent's Park
London NW1 4RG

Registered Charity No. 213280

RCOG Press Editor: Jane Moody
Design & typesetting: Tony Crowley
Printed by Latimer Trend & Co. Ltd, Estover Road, Plymouth, Devon PL6 7PY UK.
DVD produced by The Lynic Group

Contents

About the authors

Khaled M Khaled LMSSA, FRCOG, PhD
Consultant Obstetrician and Gynaecologist
Department of Obstetrics and Gynaecology
Essex Rivers Health Care Trust
Constable Wing
Turner Road
Colchester
CO4 5JL

Roopa Nair MRCOG
Specialist Registrar
Department of Obstetrics and Gynaecology
Essex Rivers Health Care Trust
Constable Wing
Turner Road
Colchester
CO4 5JL

Barry Whitlow MD, MRCOG
Consultant Obstetrician and Gynaecologist
Department of Obstetrics and Gynaecology
Essex Rivers Health Care Trust
Constable Wing
Turner Road
Colchester
CO4 5JL

Foreword

By passing the written section of the MRCOG Part Two examination, candidates demonstrate their theoretical knowledge of obstetrics and gynaecology. A large number of candidates will fail the practical (OSCE) part of the examination because they cannot apply this knowledge to clinical practice in the UK. The purpose of this book and accompanying DVD is to provide crucial tips on how to pass the Part Two OSCE section of the MRCOG examination. We have carefully selected topics that are commonly asked in the examination and have included a section on how to deal with difficult generic OSCE questions that can often throw many a good candidate.

As for any examination, it is not only important to have an in-depth knowledge of your subject and have this knowledge up-to-date by careful revision, in the OSCE examination it is also important that you can impart to the examiner and the patient (actor) the information you already know. The best practice for this is obviously clinical experience with patients and obtaining tips on how to impart such information from senior colleagues and well-run courses.

It is important that preparation for the OSCE examination is meticulous and comprehensive. The Part Two syllabus for the examination is published by the RCOG and each candidate should be fully acquainted with this syllabus. Just as for the written examination, it is vital that the candidate reads the question not just once but twice or three times before attempting to answer the question, to make sure that they follow the instructions to the letter. Some questions may involve actors and may involve difficult clinical scenarios and this can sometimes result in the candidate being distracted from subsequent questions on the OSCE circuit. It is crucial that the candidate makes a fresh start on each OSCE question, even if a previous station has been difficult, and to this end we have included a section on how to deal with such difficult OSCE stations.

We would like to extend our heartfelt thanks and sincere gratitude to all those who have given advice, help and support in the making of this pocket book and DVD. This includes our consultant colleagues at Colchester, Colin Hughes from the Computer Aided Learning Department, administrative support staff and specialist registrars who have passed the MRCOG recently (especially our gold-medal winning specialist registrar, Roopa Nair). Good luck!

Khaled Khaled
Barry Whitlow
January 2006

Khaled M Khaled, Roopa Nair and Barry Whitlow

Difficult OSCE stations

Complaint/confrontation stations

Possible scenarios:

- Angry patient
- Angry partner or relative

What sort of questions/threats to expect:

- How many have you done?
- Why was a more senior person not doing it?
- I was not told that this could happen.
- I am going to sue you.
- I am going to the media/TV.
- I will get you struck off/report you to the General Medical Council.
- I will threaten you with violence.
- I will shout/raise my voice to you.
- So you are not to blame but your colleague was negligent, wasn't he?
- I want compensation – how much is it worth?
- Why was I not given an information leaflet on this before the procedure?
- What are you going to do about it now?
- I am not satisfied with your explanation.
- You don't know what you're talking about!

How to answer

- Be firm but non-aggressive.
- Keep an open posture but do not allow yourself to be bullied.
- Explain without using medical jargon what happened and why (if possible).
- It is the patient's right if they want to take things further and you advise them that their next step would be to contact the chief executive of the trust or the complaints officer.
- If they wish to seek legal advice, that is also their right.

- They can go to the media or television if they wish, although you should not talk to such people unless directed by your defence organisation, trust press office or trust solicitor.
- They can lodge a complaint with the GMC/affiliated body if they wish – they can obtain your number from the trust if they so desire.
- If they shout, try to stay calm, with an open posture. Do not argue. Say that you can empathise with their predicament and offer the correct lines of contact if they are not satisfied with your explanation (patient advice and liaison service or chief executive).
- Do not implicate colleagues, even if you think they are to blame – that is for an independent review panel to decide.
- Do not give any cash figures as to what compensation they are entitled to, if any – again that is for the courts to decide, if indeed liability is proven.
- If no leaflet given, it is not necessarily department protocol to provide one and the individual doctor concerned with consenting the patient should decide whether you require additional information.
- Suggest patient advice and liaison service.

Briefly explain the complaints procedure:

1. Letter to chief executive.
2. Meeting with consultant concerned and/or department managers with or without the chief executive.
3. Independent review panel.
4. Settle out of court.
5. Settle in court.
6. GMC hearing/action.

Breaking bad news stations

These may involve diagnosis of cancer, intrauterine death or miscarriage.

- Speak clearly.
- Maintain good eye contact.
- Break the news in a stepwise fashion.

Domestic violence station

Domestic violence is an important issue in current practice. You must be aware of this. Make sure that you are aware of the essential aspects of this issue before the examination by asking a senior colleague.

How to use the DVD

All candidates sitting the OSCE examination should be prepared to deal with certain difficult scenarios.

You will often encounter a role player in the OSCE examination, who plays the part of a patient in distress or in a confrontational situation. The OSCE is no different from the clinic, where registrars see their patients in the hospital atmosphere. If the candidate confines him or herself to that atmosphere they will have the best chance of passing.

The DVD enclosed with this book covers life scenarios that are all of paramount importance in clinical practice. The cases were selected from the most difficult scenarios possible, where experience cannot be gained except by watching these stations.

We appreciate that this is a very small part of the examination but such stations are designed to test the ability of the candidate to deal with difficult situations – and practice makes perfect.

We suggest that before you play the DVD you seek the advice of a senior colleague in your department who could help you or alternatively, ask a colleague and try to role play the scenario in the station before you watch it.

It may be useful if you make notes. This could help to improve your performance and identify your weaknesses.

The DVD cannot cover all the cases we would like to include but we hope that it gives you just an idea of the kinds of situations that you might encounter. We hope that you will be able to build on this to develop your own style.

Station 1

You are the registrar in clinic and are seeing Mrs B, who is
35 years of age. She complains of worsening periods over the past 2 years.
You are required to take an appropriate history and discuss management
options with her.

Examination findings will be provided.

Marks will be awarded for:

- introduction and appropriate eye contact
- listening to the patient and answering her questions
- taking a history – symptoms – onset and duration:
  - intermenstrual and postcoital bleeding
  - dysmenorrhoea/dyspareunia
  - previous menstrual patterns
  - obstetric history
  - contraception/smear
  - medical history
  - surgical history
  - drugs and allergies – including treatment for periods
  - smoking.

Examination reveals a 24-week sized mass with irregular contour, suggestive
of fibroids.

Investigations:

- Full blood count
- Ultrasound scan
- Hormonal investigations not indicated
- Appropriate explanation of tests to patient.

Treatment options explained to patient:

- Conservative
- Surgical:
  - myomectomy
  - uterine artery embolisation
  - hysterectomy
- Medical:
  - gonadotrophin-releasing hormone analogues ⎫
  - danazols   ⎬ short term
  - tranexamic/mefenamic acid: may not be fully effective
  - hormonal: may not be fully effective

Station 2

This is a structured viva. The examiner will ask you some questions.

A 38-year-old woman attends your gynaecology clinic requesting reversal of sterilisation.

Q. How will you approach this patient?

Answer:

- Sympathetic and understanding approach
- Reason for reversal explored
- Type of sterilisation if known
- Interval since sterilisation
- Obstetric history
- Counsel re:
  - lack of availability on NHS
  - success rate
  - need for investigations prior to decision.

Q. What factors related to the sterilisation could affect success rate?

Answer:

- Type of sterilisation – success rate best with clips, least with diathermy or excision.
- Interval since sterilisation – longer interval associated with lower success.
- Length of fallopian tube left – success rate lower if less than 4 cm.
- Area of tube to be reanastomosed – isthmo-isthmic has best prognosis.

Khaled M Khaled, Roopa Nair and Barry Whitlow

Q. What investigations would be performed before reversal?

Answer:

- Semen analysis.
- Assessment of ovulation.
- Laparoscopy:
  - to judge length of tube
  - co-morbidities such as pelvic adhesions or endometriosis, which reduce success.

Q. What are the success rates for the procedure?

Answer:

Success rates vary with type of procedure and operator experience. In good hands and with microsurgical techniques, rates of 75–80% may be achieved.

Station 3

Mrs Elder, a 38-year-old primigravida who is 16 weeks pregnant, is scheduled for amniocentesis. Down syndrome screening revealed a high risk of 1:8. Obtain her consent for the procedure.

Marks will be awarded for:

- appropriate introduction and eye contact
- avoiding medical jargon
- explaining the high-risk result and reason for amniocentesis
- exploring the patient's wishes if amniocentesis reveals Down syndrome
- checking whether patient understands
- explaining details of procedure
- complications, including risk of miscarriage
- results – fluorescence in situ hybridisation available in 48 hours, detailed around 2–3 weeks
- inviting questions and responding appropriately
- obtaining signature on consent form.

Khaled M Khaled, Roopa Nair and Barry Whitlow

Station 4

This is a structured viva. The examiner will ask you some questions.

You are called to the accident and emergency department to see 28-year-old Mary Bloom, who is complaining of severe abdominal pain. She has been receiving fertility treatment and has had two embryos transferred 23 days ago.

Q. What is the most likely diagnosis?

Answer:

- Ectopic pregnancy.
- Ovarian hyperstimulation syndrome (OHSS).

Q. What are the risk factors for OHSS?

Answer:

- Young age.
- Low body mass index.
- Polycystic ovaries.
- Use of gonadotrophins.
- Previous OHSS.
- Large number of follicles.
- Pregnancy.

Q. What investigations would you perform?

Answer:

- Blood investigations:
  - full blood count – white blood cells and packed cell volume (haemoconcentration)
  - clotting screen
  - creatinine
  - urea and electrolyes – for hyponatraemia and hyperkalaemia
  - liver function tests

- ◆ albumin levels.
- Chest X-ray
- Ultrasound scan – ovarian size.

Q. What would be your management?

Answer:

Conservative management:

- admission – high-dependency or intensive care unit if severe
- intravenous rehydration
- analgesics
- thromboprophylaxis – thromboembolic stockings, heparin
- symptomatic relief of vomiting
- monitoring of parameters including vital signs, central venous pressure, abdominal girth, daily weight, urine output, blood chemistry
- paracentesis/pleural tap/dialysis
- albumin infusion.

Diuretics should not be used.

In severe cases, termination of pregnancy.

Q. How would OHSS be prevented?

Answer:

- Identification of risk factors
- Use of alternative methods of ovulation induction (ovarian drilling, clomifene)
- Avoiding downregulation
- Use of pure follicle-stimulating hormone
- Cycle cancellation/oocyte aspiration and cryopreservation of embryos
- Progesterone rather than human chorionic gonadotrophin for luteal phase support.

Station 5

You receive a telephone call from Dr Smith, a GP, regarding an antenatal patient Barbara Jones. You are expected to carry out a telephone consultation with him.

Dr Smith: Good morning, Dr. X, I am Dr Smith, a general practitioner.

You: Good morning, I am Dr. X, registrar on call. How can I help you?

Dr Smith: I was wondering if you could give me some advice please.

You: Sure.

Dr Smith: I have with me Mrs Barbara Jones, who is 28 weeks into her first pregnancy. She complained of vaginal discharge and I took some swabs. They grew group B streptococcus (GBS). What should I do?

You: Is she symptomatic at present?

Dr Smith: No, the discharge has cleared.

You: Have we recently performed a midstream urine test?

Dr Smith: Yes, and it was clear.

You: Well, in the absence of bacteruria and in an asymptomatic patient, by the Royal College guidelines, antenatal treatment is not needed.

Dr Smith: What if any of those are present?

You: Treatment with phenoxymethylpenicillin (penicillin V) four times daily for 7 days would be indicated.

Dr Smith: So, can she be reassured?

You: Yes, but she will need antibiotic prophylaxis in labour.

Dr Smith: What prophylaxis?

You: Benzylpenicillin intravenously 4-hourly or clindamycin if she is allergic to penicillin.

Dr Smith: Would the baby need treatment as well?

You: The paediatricians would be informed and the baby would have swabs.

Dr Smith: How dangerous is GBS?

You: Well, although found in 25–30% of women, around 1 in 1000 babies can have severe septicaemia or meningitis, leading to death.

Dr Smith: In that case, why do we not screen all women?

You: It has been found that because of the low incidence of neonatal disease, routine screening is not cost effective. A risk factor-based approach is recommended. At-risk pregnancies including:

- previous neonatal GBS
- GBS bacteria
- premature rupture of the membranes
- preterm labour
- intrapartum pyrexia.

Dr Smith: Well that was educational. Thank you very much.

You: Thank you.

Station 6

Miss Sindu, who is a known carrier of the beta-thalassaemia trait, wishes to start a family. She is anxious about the implications of her condition on the pregnancy. Counsel her.

Marks will be awarded for:

- appropriate introduction and eye contact
- understanding patient's anxiety
- responding to questions appropriately
- sympathetic and reassuring approach
- partner screening if also carrier, then one in four chance of having baby with thalassaemia major
- implications of beta-thalassaemia:
  - anaemia
  - diabetes
  - hepatic cirrhosis
  - cardiomyopathy
  - death
- availability of prenatal techniques to detect this condition
- option of termination if baby is affected
- importance of screening both partners for other haemoglobinopathies, such as sickle cell
- increased folic acid requirements, therefore advice regarding supplementation.

Station 7

You are the registrar on call and are reviewing Miss Hicks, a 24-year-old woman, 2 weeks after suction evacuation for an incomplete miscarriage. The histology report is suggestive of complete mole. Discuss the report with her.

Marks will be awarded for:

- appropriate introduction, eye contact and avoiding medical jargon
- sensitive approach
- explaining clearly the histology report in simple terms
- avoiding use of the word cancer at this point
- stressing the importance of follow up
- registration with regional trophoblastic centre
- monitoring of serum and urinary beta human chorionic gonadotrophin
- chemotherapy if levels are high (only if patient asks)
- contraceptive advice
- inviting questions and responding appropriately.

Khaled M Khaled, Roopa Nair and Barry Whitlow

Station 8

You are asked to counsel Miss Higgins, a 38-year-old nulliparous teacher, who requests prophylactic oophorectomy. Her mother died of ovarian cancer at 40 years of age.

Marks will be awarded for:

- appropriate introduction and eye contact
- use of non-medical language
- understanding patient's anxiety
- most ovarian cancer non-hereditary (less than 5% genetic)
- explores patient's family history – high risk/low risk
- genetics centre referral if high risk
- *BRCA1* – screening offered
- screening methods – serum CA125 and transvaginal sonography
- limitations of screening, UK Collaborative Trial of Ovarian Cancer Screening for low-risk population (only for women over 50 years of age)
- prophylactic oophorectomy does not eliminate risk
- chemoprophylaxis – role of combined oral contraceptive in prevention.

Station 9

You are seeing Mr Brown in the fertility clinic. Mr and Mrs Brown have been together for 6 years and have been trying to conceive for 4 years. Mrs Brown has one child by a previous relationship. Mr Brown's semen result is as shown (result showing azoospermia). Your task is to discuss further management with Mr Brown.

Marks will be awarded for:

- appropriate greeting and eye contact
- obtaining history:
  - mumps
  - orchitis
  - chemo/radiotherapy
  - testicular/inguinal surgery
  - drugs – androgens/steroids
  - medical illnesses – diabetes
  - occupation
  - smoking
  - tight underpants
- explaining need for examination and investigations after explaining semen result
- brief history of female partner
- need for investigation of ovulation and tubal patency
- repeat semen analysis, follicle-stimulating hormone, luteinising hormone, testicular biopsy and karyotype
- management of testicular causes: intracytoplasmic sperm injection (ICSI)/donor insemination
- management of post-testicular causes: surgical treatment, ICSI
- inviting questions
- avoiding medical jargon.

Khaled M Khaled, Roopa Nair and Barry Whitlow

Station 10

You are shown an intrauterine contraceptive device. Discuss it with the examiner.

Marks will be awarded for:

- identification of the intrauterine contraceptive device (Mirena®)
- levonorgestrel-containing, releases 52 micrograms/day
- discussion of mechanism of action
- effective for 5 years
- contraceptive effectiveness
- indications
- contraindications
- adverse effects
- non-contraceptive uses:
  - menorrhagia 86% reduction in mean blood loss in 6 months and 97% after 1 year
  - endometriosis
  - dysmenorrhoea
  - fibroids
  - progestogen arm of hormone replacement therapy
- complications of insertion:
  - infection
  - uterine perforation
  - expulsion
  - bleeding abnormalities.

Station 11

After a routine total abdominal hysterectomy and bilateral salpingo-oophorectomy, Mrs Jones was ready for discharge when she noticed a leak of clear fluid from her vagina. You are the registrar on call and have been called to see her. The examiner will ask you some questions.

Q. What will be your first steps?

Answer:

- Review operative notes for preoperative risk factors and any intraoperative difficulties.
- History and examination.

Q. Examination reveals pooling of urine in the vagina. What would be your next steps?

Answer:

- Sympathetic approach to patient, express regret.
- Keep her informed of possibility of bladder injury.
- Catheter, midstream urine.
- Inform operating surgeon.
- Organise cystoscopy and intravenous urography.
- Urologist referral.

Q. Cystoscopy and IVU reveal a vesicovaginal fistula near the trigone. What further management would be necessary?

Answer:

- Allow oedema and infection to settle.
- Small fistulas may heal with catheterisation.
- Definitive repair – urologists.
- Debriefing and counselling of patient.
- Helping her to cope and explaining further management plans.

Khaled M Khaled, Roopa Nair and Barry Whitlow

Q. Principles of fistula repair?

Answer:

- Absorbable suture.
- Elliptical incision, wide mobilisation, repair without tension.
- Watertight closure.
- Timing 10–12 weeks postoperatively.

Station 12

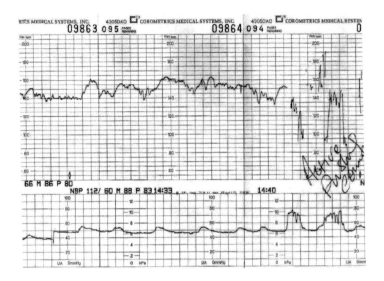

Interpret the CTG (above): G2P1, 38 weeks, ruptured membranes, fully dilated, meconium-stained liquor.

Marks will be awarded for:

- noting time on CTG
- paper speed
- contractions – comment
- all components to be described:
  - baseline (reassuring/nonreassuring)
  - variability
  - accelerations
  - decelerations – early, late, variable (typical/atypical)
- overall impression:
  - normal
  - suspicious
  - pathological
- measures to be taken.

Station 13

A 76-year-old woman presents with a lump "down below" for 6 weeks. You are seeing her in clinic. Examination findings will be provided.

Marks will be awarded for:

- appropriate introduction and eye contact
- history:
  - nature of lump
  - increase in size
  - pruritus
  - bleeding, bowel, urinary problems
  - weight
  - smoking
  - medical history
  - family history.

Examination reveals a hard, indurated cauliflower-like growth 0.5 cm diameter on the vulva.

Discuss investigations:

- full blood count
- general anaesthetic fitness
- excisional biopsy (full marks only if excisional explained)
- management depending on histology.

Marks will be awarded for:

- inviting questions, responding appropriately
- not using word cancer in first instance
- follow-up appointment.

Station 14

You are asked to counsel a woman for HIV testing. Miss Shaw is 32 years of age and is 12 weeks pregnant. She was a known drug abuser but has now stopped. She has had multiple sexual partners. She is unsure about undergoing testing.

Marks will be awarded for:

- sympathetic approach
- non-judgmental attitude
- sensitive handling of high-risk status
- non-biased information about HIV
- avoiding medical jargon
- benefits of testing in pregnancy:
  - reduces vertical transmission to less than 2%
  - antiretrovirals
  - caesarean section
  - avoidance of breastfeeding
- benefits of treatment to woman, if she is positive
- poor prognosis for children infected – 50% die by 1 year
- leaving decision to patient, assuring her that declining testing will not affect her care
- follow-up appointment.

Station 15

You are seeing Mrs Baker in the prepregnancy clinic for counselling. Mrs Baker is a known epileptic on sodium valproate. Her first pregnancy was terminated at 12 weeks for anencephaly. Her last fit was 2 months ago.

Marks will be awarded for:

- appropriate introduction and eye contact
- avoiding medical jargon
- advising optimal seizure control and drug regimen (liaison with neurologist) before planning pregnancy
- preconceptual folic acid for 3 months (5 mg dose)
- effects of antiepileptic drugs (valproate) on fetus:
  - neural tube defects
  - craniofacial abnormalities
- emphasising need to continue drug
- reassurance
- inviting questions
- detailed fetal ultrasound and maternal alphafetoprotein levels
- surveillance during pregnancy – growth scans
- follow-up appointment.

Station 16

This is a structured viva. The examiner will ask you some questions.

Q. What are GNRH agonists?

Answer:

- They are synthetised by substitution of amino acids in the gonadotrophin-releasing hormone (GNRH) molecule. This leads to increased duration of action.
- Initial flare effect.
- Downregulation of pituitary receptors leading to a hypogonadotrophic state.

Q. Discuss their various uses.

Answer:

- Endometriosis.
- Preoperative – fibroids.
- Infertility – induction of ovulation (discuss protocols).

Q. What is the role of addback therapy?

Answer:

- Preoperative.
- Endometriosis.
- Premenstrual syndrome.

Q. What preparations are available?

Answer:

- Leuprorelin acetate.
- Goserelin.
- Nafarelin.

Khaled M Khaled, Roopa Nair and Barry Whitlow

Station 17

You are asked to see Mrs Day, a 35-year-old primigravida with 6 weeks amenorrhoea and a positive pregnancy test. She complains of spotting over the past week. Ultrasound reveals a gestational sac of 19 mm with no fetal pole. Explain the scan findings and management plan.

Marks will be awarded for:

- introduction and eye contact
- avoiding medical jargon
- sympathetic approach
- explaining correct diagnosis and management – does not fit criteria for miscarriage, therefore rescan after 1 week
- listening to patient
- inviting questions and responding appropriately
- discussing management of miscarriage only if asked by patient
- conservative
- medical: mifepristone and misoprostol
- surgical evacuation.

Station 18

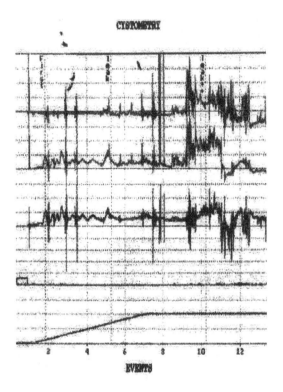

CYSTOMETRY

EVENTS

You are given the urodynamic test report of 52-year-old Mrs Lewis (above), who complains of worsening leakage of urine on coughing and straining. She also complains of urgency and frequency. You are asked to interpret the report and outline management options to the examiner.

Marks will be awarded for:

- correctly describing the various graphs:
    - Pabd – abdominal pressure (cm H_2O)
    - Pves – bladder pressure (cm H_2O)
    - Pdet – detrusor pressure (obtained by subtracting Pabd from Pves)
    - Qura – rate of flow (ml/second)
    - Vinf – volume infused (ml)

Khaled M Khaled, Roopa Nair and Barry Whitlow

- describing the following:
  - filling phase
  - provocative tests
  - pressure flow studies (voiding)
- correct diagnosis – detrusor instability
- normal values (if asked by examiner):
  - first urge 150–200 ml
  - residual urine less than 50 ml
  - peak flow rate greater than 15 ml/second
  - no detrusor pressure rise on filling
  - detrusor pressure rise less than 50 cm H_2O on voiding
- management options for detrusor instability:
  - conservative – lifestyle modifications, bladder training, anticholinergics: oxybutynin, tolterodine, trospium, solifenacin
  - surgical – clam ileocystoplasty.

Station 19

You are asked to see a 50-year-old woman who has been admitted for surgery for urodynamic stress incontinence. She has opted to undergo a transvaginal tape insertion. Obtain consent for operation after discussing the relevant issues with her.

Marks will be awarded for:

- appropriate greeting, introduction and eye contact
- avoiding medical jargon
- explaining procedure in simple language:
  - local anaesthesia and sedation/general anaesthesia/spinal anaesthesia
  - suprapubic and vaginal incisions
  - insertion of tape
  - cystoscopy
- success rate 80–90%, symptoms better in over 90%
- risks:
  - bladder perforation
  - bleeding
  - abdominal bruising
  - urinary infection
- postoperative problems:
  - postoperative voiding difficulty
  - worsening of symptoms
  - wound infection
  - urinary infection
  - erosion of tape
- anaesthetic risks
- checking whether patient has understood
- inviting questions and responding appropriately
- obtaining signature on consent form.

Khaled M Khaled, Roopa Nair and Barry Whitlow

Station 20

You are asked to see a 34-year-old African Caribbean woman who is 18 weeks pregnant and has come for her booking visit. She is known to smoke and to use heroin, and she has recently been started on methadone. Counsel her regarding her antenatal care.

Marks will be awarded for:

- identifying risk factors (smoking, heroin use)
- adopting a non-judgemental attitude
- holistic approach with multidisciplinary input (including social workers and liaison with drug authority)
- screening for sexually transmitted infections, HIV, hepatitis B and C
- explaining effects of smoking:
  - intrauterine growth restriction
  - perinatal morbidity
  - bleeding
  - premature rupture of the membranes
  - sudden infant death syndrome
- explaining effects of heroin:
  - antepartum haemorrhage
  - premature rupture of the membranes
  - preterm labour
  - intrauterine growth restriction
  - perinatal morbidity and mortality
  - neonatal withdrawal
- NHS smoking helpline
- consultant-led care
- antenatal visits
- ultrasound scan
- paediatric involvement
- child protection issues.

Station 21

You are the on-call registrar for the labour ward and have been called to a room where a multigravid woman is in the second stage of labour. The head has delivered and the midwife is experiencing difficulty in delivering the shoulders.

Marks will be awarded for:

- call for help – SHO, anaesthetist, operating department practitioner, senior midwife and paediatrician
- episiotomy – evaluate
- McRoberts' manoeuvre, suprapubic pressure, Rubin II, Wood's screw, Wood's reverse screw, delivery of posterior arm, all-fours position
- additional – Zavanelli, symphysiotomy, cleidotomy
- management of team
- management of the third stage
- risk management – documentation
- debriefing
- follow up baby
- next delivery, glucose tolerance test prior to discharge.

Khaled M Khaled, Roopa Nair and Barry Whitlow

Station 22

You are the registrar on call for the labour ward. At 3 a.m. the emergency buzzer goes off and the midwife calls, "Patient bleeding". You rush to the room and see a recently delivered woman with a pool of blood beneath her. The midwife is rubbing up a contraction. What steps would you take?

Marks will be awarded for:

- immediate actions:
  - call for help
  - summon appropriate staff – anaesthetist, operating department practitioner, midwives, senior house officer
  - estimate blood loss
  - activate local massive haemorrhage protocol
- check A, B, C, large-bore cannulae, fluids, O_2
- rub up contraction
- empty bladder – catheter
- check placenta whether delivered and complete
- bloods for investigation and crossmatching
- inform duty consultant
- bimanual compression
- drugs – Syntometrine, oxytocin, carboprost
- allocate one midwife for baby and partner
- theatre, check for trauma
- possible operative interventions
- blood and blood products
- after bleeding controlled:
  - high-dependency unit
  - antibiotics
  - thromboprophylaxis
  - debriefing and counselling
  - risk management reporting.

Station 23

You are the consultant obstetrician about to see Mr Alexander, whose wife was under your care during her pregnancy. During the second stage, decelerations were noted for which an instrumental delivery was undertaken. However, the baby was stillborn. The husband is angry and has demanded an appointment to see you. Postmortem examination was unhelpful.

Marks will be awarded for:

- appropriate introduction and eye contact
- sympathetic approach
- expressing regret and sympathy
- enquiring about wellbeing of his wife
- not interrupting husband
- not reacting aggressively
- offering counselling
- not blaming colleagues
- explaining postmortem findings in suitable language
- explaining complaints procedure.

Khaled M Khaled, Roopa Nair and Barry Whitlow

Station 24

You are the consultant in charge. You have recently operated on a 42-year-old woman with abdominal pain and menorrhagia, with ultrasound appearances suggestive of an endometriotic/dermoid cyst. A total abdominal hysterectomy and bilateral salpingo-oophorectomy was performed at the time. The histopathology has revealed mucinous cystadenocarcinoma of both ovaries. You are about to break this news to her.

Marks will be awarded for:

- appropriate greeting and eye contact
- checking whether patient is alone or has a relative
- appropriate discussion and explanation of diagnosis
- expressing regret
- giving patient time
- acknowledging shock
- offering future meetings
- outlining management plan
- arranging follow-up visit and nursing support
- overall empathy, kindness and support.

Station 25

You are the senior registrar and have been asked to see a couple in their first pregnancy. A 20-week scan has revealed anencephaly. A 12-week scan had been performed elsewhere. The couple are extremely distressed and angry.

Marks will be awarded for:

- appropriate introduction
- expressing regret and sympathy
- acknowledging couple's shock and anger
- staying calm and sympathetic
- responding to questions
- offering options for further management
- offering counselling
- next pregnancy issues
- low recurrence risk
- offering follow-up visit.

Khaled M Khaled, Roopa Nair and Barry Whitlow

Station 26

You are the consultant in charge. You have recently operated on Mrs Xavier, aged 40 years, and had performed a total abdominal hysterectomy for severe endometriosis. At the time of surgery, bowel injury was noted. A colostomy was performed and the injury was repaired by the general surgeons. You are now conducting a postoperative clinic visit.

Marks will be awarded for:

- appropriate greeting and eye contact
- listening to patient and inviting questions
- expressing sympathy and regret
- sympathetic approach
- explaining accidental bowel damage
- asking about other problems and wellbeing
- colostomy care
- arrangements at home
- explaining plans for further management
- offering follow-up visit.

Station 27

You are the registrar on call taking a delivery suite handover at 0830 hours. You have with you an obstetric SHO with 3 months' experience, a second-year anaesthetic SpR and six midwives. IL, AR and ES can secure IV lines. DK has no specific skills. The on-call consultant is available but is doing an interview session. You decide what tasks are needed, in what order and to whom they should be allocated.

Room	Name	GP	Gestation	Liquor	Epidural	Synto	Comments	Midwife
1	AB1	P1	33 weeks	–	–	No	Post LSCS; 1200 ml blood loss; baby on SCBU	IL
2	CD2	P4	41 weeks	Clear	Yes	No	7 cm dilated at 3 a.m.	MH
3	EF3	P0	28 weeks	–	–	–	tightening loin pain	DK
4	GH4	P0	21 weeks	–	–	–	Termination for fetal anomaly; misoprostol received 2100 hours last night	IL
5	IJ5	P1	39 weeks	Meconium-stained	Yes	Yes	VBAC 5 cm at 0300 hours, 6 cm at 0700 hours	AR
6	KL6	P8	40 weeks	Clear	No	No	Fully dilated; urge to push	ES
7	MN7	P0	34 weeks	–	–	–	Complete placenta praevia; tightening; bleeding	HG
8	OP8	P2	41 weeks	–	–	–	Delivered at 0745; episiotomy needs suturing	ES

Delivery Suite Board

Marks will be awarded for:

Tasks to be performed:

Room 1   Review pulse, blood pressure, input/output chart, blood loss. Repeat FBC, clotting. Check drugs, IV fluids, condition of baby.

Room 2   Needs assessment by doctor. CTG? Oxytocin.

Room 3   Needs assessment and CTG.

Room 4   Reassessment for further misoprostol.

Room 5   Needs assessment for progress and CTG. Check FBC, group and save.

Room 6   Check IV line, blood sent. Active management of third stage.

Room 7   Needs urgent assessment. Bloods for FBC, crossmatch. Inform special care baby unit. CTG. Needs consultant input. Senior anaesthetist.

Room 8   Needs suturing.

Priority of tasks and allocation of duties:

- urgent registrar review in rooms 7, 5 and 2
- semi-urgent review room 4
- SHO to assess room 3
- anaesthetist and SHO to review room 1 – routine
- anaesthetist to see room 7 urgently
- midwife to suture room 8
- senior midwife to supervise room 6.

Station 28

You are presented with a gynaecology theatre waiting list. You are expected to decide what is the appropriate operation for the patient, the venue (inpatient etc.), priority (urgent, soon or routine) and any special needs. You will discuss this with the examiner at the next station.

1. 62 years   P0 + 0 virgo intacta
   History of hypertension and diabetes, recurrent post-menopausal bleeding
   Family history of ovarian cancer

2. 40 years   Deep dyspareunia
   Menorrhagia, ovarian cyst greater than 8 cm

3. 18 years   Small ulcer on right labia majora
   Urinary retention

4. 78 years   Vulval itching
   Small ulcer on right labia, inguinal glands enlarged

5. 29 years   Apareunia, painful episiotomy
   Breastfeeding. 10/52 postnatal

Answer:

1. High risk for endometrial cancer. Hysteroscopy and curettage – inpatient. Urgent. Needs ultrasound, anaesthetic fitness.

2. Possible endometriosis. Laparoscopic ovarian cystectomy as inpatient. Soon. Needs ultrasound and serum CA125. Also important to know history of previous surgeries and family history.

3. Possible herpes. Does not need surgery. Swabs and referral to GUM clinic. Symptomatic treatment.

4. Rise of vulva cancer – needs urgent excisional biopsy as day case. May need referral to cancer centre.

5. Possible atrophic vagina due to breastfeeding. See in clinic after breastfeeding stopped. Try interim lubricants. If persistent may need perineal refashioning – routine day case.

Station 29

You are asked to conduct a preoperative ward round. The patients on the list are:

1. Vaginal hysterectomy. Mrs X. Age 48 years.
2. Laparoscopic sterilisation. Mrs W. Age 32 years.
3. Resection of submucosal fibroid. Mrs Y. Age 35 years.

You will be asked a few questions.

Q. Regarding Mrs X, what would you do on your round?

Answer:

- Read through previous medical notes.
- Check that she understands the operation.
- Check that she still has symptoms and wishes to go ahead.
- Discuss success rates.
- Discuss complications.
- Check smear history, rule out pregnancy.
- Send Hb, group and save.
- Consent.

Q. What further pre- and postoperative practical measures would be taken?

Answer:

- See anaesthetist.
- Sign consent form.
- Antibiotics, thromboprophylaxis.
- Intravenous fluids.
- Catheter – urinary.
- Pain relief.
- Early mobilisation.

What would you discuss with Mrs W?

Answer:

- Check whether she understands the procedure.
- Ask for LMP, rule out pregnancy.
- Ask for history of previous abdominal surgeries.
- Explain that sterilisation is irreversible.
- Explain failure rate 1/200.
- Increased risk of ectopic pregnancy.
- Risk of bowel and major vessel injury with risk of laparotomy.
- Discuss other alternative methods.
- Need to use contraception till next period.
- Day case surgery.
- Would need someone to drive her home and take care of her overnight.
- Consent form.

What issues would you discuss with Mrs Y?

Answer:

- Check whether she understands procedure.
- Ask for LMP, rule out pregnancy.
- Discuss procedure and success rate.
- Discuss complications.
- Check whether endometrium has been prepared-GnRH analogues, danazol.
- Need for further follow up in case of infertility.
- Consent form.

Station 30

Critically appraise a patient information leaflet given to you.

Answer:

- Author of leaflet, topic, date of review, for whom.
- Layout, presentation.
- Content and subject matter.
- Positive points.
- Negative points.
- Medical jargon, language, diagrams.
- Value of leaflets for patients.
- Different languages for ethnic groups.
- Dissemination of leaflet.
- Other sources of information for patient.

Station 31

You were the third-year specialist registrar on call and had delivered a baby by ventouse delivery for prolonged second stage. The delivery was uncomplicated but the baby developed Erb's palsy.

Write a risk management report.

Answer:

- If any adverse event, preliminary reports must be recorded.
- Report to clinical director.
- Record name, designation and signature, experience and competence.
- Names, status and role of staff involved.
- Discuss whether antenatal and intrapartum care appropriate.
- Documentation of events.
- Indications for assisted delivery.
- Any factor that could alter outcome.
- Was shoulder dystocia present.
- Factual description of events.

Khaled M Khaled, Roopa Nair and Barry Whitlow

Station 32

How would you conduct an audit on admissions in your hospital to the intensive care unit from our specialty.

Answer:

- Describe the audit cycle.
- Retrospective/prospective.
- Sample size?
- Review criteria, target levels.
- Pro forma, data collection (including missing data).
- Data analysis.
- Review results.
- Recommendations and feedback to staff.
- Modify practice – changes in protocols/departmental organisation.
- Re-audit after reasonable period.

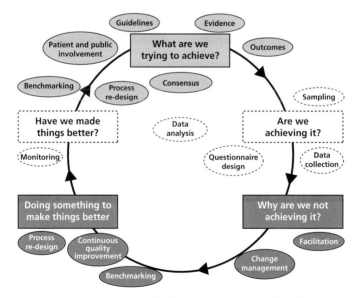

The clinical audit cycle; (reproduced with permission from RCOG Clinical Governance Advice No. 5: Understanding audit. 2003; www.rcog.org.uk/index.asp?PageID=476)

Station 33

Draw up a protocol to reduce the incidence of wound infections in your hospital.

Answer:

- Importance of topic.
- Benchmarking – literature search/RCOG guidelines.
- Identify risk factors for wound infection.
- Identify resource implications.
- Form a group involving stakeholders.
- Make protocol (including preoperative/intraoperative/postoperative).
- Implementation.
- Potential difficulties and solutions.
- Multidisciplinary feedback.
- Audit.

 Khaled M Khaled, Roopa Nair and Barry Whitlow

Station 34

You are presented with details of a 34-year-old G2P1 at 30 weeks with confirmed spontaneous rupture of the membranes. Her previous obstetric and medical history is uncomplicated. You will have a viva with the examiner.

Q. What are the risks of preterm prelabour rupture of the membranes?

Answer:

- Maternal:
  - preterm labour
  - chorioamnionitis and septicaemia
  - risk of operative interventions
  - malpresentations
- Fetal:
  - cord prolapse
  - prematurity – respiratory distress syndrome, chronic lung disease, necrotising enterocolitis, intraventricular haemorrhage, feeding problems
  - group B streptococcal infection
  - cerebral palsy

Q. What drugs would you use and what is the evidence base?

Answer:

- Steroids – betamethasone, dexamethasone (RCOG)
- Antibiotics – erythromycin (ORACLE)
- Tocolytics – when, which drugs

Q. What factors would determine timing of delivery?

Answer:

- Features of chorioamnionitis
- 36 weeks if conservative treatment

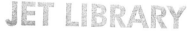

Q. If caesarean section at 30 weeks, what incisions?

Answer:

- Low transverse
- Classical – safer for baby
- J-shaped

Station 35

You are seeing 25-year-old Tina Wakeley in the gynaecology clinic. She gave birth to her fourth child 3 months ago and is not breastfeeding. She believes that no contraceptive method is reliable and requests a hysterectomy, as she is certain she does not want any more children. You are required to talk to her.

Marks will be awarded for:

- appropriate introduction and eye contact
- sensitive and firm handling of request for hysterectomy
- listening to patient's concerns
- persuading patient to consider options
- barrier methods
- oral contraceptive pills/minipill/Implanon®/Depo Provera®
- Mirena®/other intrauterine contraceptive devices
- female sterilisation/vasectomy
- helping patient arrive at decision
- offering follow-up appointment.

Station 36

Mrs Douglas has been referred by her midwife to discuss antenatal Down syndrome screening. Mrs Douglas is 39 years old and is very concerned about this baby. Your task is to help her decide what tests she will have.

Marks will be awarded for:

- sensitive, sympathetic approach
- advising about background risks
- explaining types of tests – screening and diagnostic
- screening tests – low-risk or high-risk results
- nuchal translucency 76%
- combined test 80%
- serum screening – second trimester 77%
- integrated test 90%
- ultrasound scan at 20 weeks – 50%
- definitive tests – chorionic villus sampling and amniocentesis – risk of miscarriage.

Station 37

You have been asked to see Mrs Jacobs in the antenatal clinic. She is 19 years of age and 20 weeks into her first pregnancy. The GP has referred her for persistent vaginal discharge. She has had four courses of antibiotics and swabs have all been negative. You are required to talk to this patient.

Marks will be awarded for:

- sympathetic approach
- discovering 'hidden agenda' such as domestic violence presenting as a nonspecific complaint of persistent vaginal discharge
- listening to the patient's problem
- non-patronising and non-judgemental approach
- not her fault
- offering to help
- access to complaints – police
- offering practical suggestions
- Women's Aid, local women's groups
- escape plan.

Station 38

You are the registrar in gynaecology clinic. You are seeing Mrs Price, who has been referred by the GP for abnormal results on a routine cervical smear. She is anxious and has many questions to ask you. Her smear test result showed moderate dyskaryosis.

Marks will be awarded for:

- appropriate introduction and eye contact
- avoiding medical jargon
- explaining results appropriately
- checking that patient understands and responding appropriately to her questions
- relation to HPV infection, 80% of women have it during lifetime
- persistence of infection related to immunity
- not cancer
- may need treatment to prevent progression
- explaining future plan including colposcopy and various treatments
- outlining need and timing of follow up
- overall reassuring and sympathetic approach.

Khaled M Khaled, Roopa Nair and Barry Whitlow

Station 39

You are seeing Mrs Davey, who delivered a stillborn baby 1 day ago. She had been admitted at 39 weeks with reduced fetal movements over 3 days; ultrasound confirmed intrauterine death. Labour was induced and a stillborn girl weighing 2.8 kg was delivered.

Marks will be awarded for:

- appropriate introduction and eye contact, sympathetic approach
- expressing sympathy and regret
- asking about physical health and family support
- encouraging mother to vent feelings
- ensuring she does not blame herself
- arranging for her to see baby, offering photographs and mementos
- discussing postmortem and other investigations sensitively
- funeral arrangements
- counselling, SANDS (Stillbirth and Neonatal Deaths Society)
- breast milk suppression
- follow-up appointment.

Station 40

You are asked to counsel a 28-year-old primigravida who is undergoing an elective caesarean section for major placenta praevia at 38 weeks. The examiner will ask you a few questions.

Q. What preoperative measures would be taken?

Answer:

- Review notes.
- Ultrasound scan – placental position.
- Counselling – preoperative, intraoperative and postoperative details.
- Consent.
- Bloods – crossmatch.
- Premedication.
- Inform anaesthetist, consultant obstetrician, consultant haematologist.
- Catheter – indwelling.
- Antibiotics.
- Thromboprophylaxis.

Q. What intraoperative measures would you take to reduce bleeding?

Answer:
- Ensure blood in theatre.
- Delivery of baby
  - cutting through placenta
  - rupture of membranes
- Syntocinon infusion.
- Stitches if bleeding from placental bed.
- Closure.
- Drain.

Q. What postoperative actions would be taken?

Answer:

- Catheter.
- Drain.
- Thromboembolic compression stockings (TEDS).
- Antibiotics, thromboprophylaxis.
- Anti D.
- Contraception and discussion of future pregnancies at postnatal visit.

Station 41

You are asked to see 39-year-old Laura Singleton, who has arrived at the maternity unit with acute abdominal pain. You are expected to take a history and discuss management options with her. Examination findings will be provided.

Marks will be awarded for:

- appropriate introduction, eye contact and nonmedical language
- obtaining relevant history:
    - primigravida
    - LMP, EDD: 26 weeks pregnant, singleton
    - current complaints
    - details of current pregnancy – scans, Down syndrome risk – amniocentesis
    - contraceptive and smear history
    - medical/surgical
    - family history
    - urinary/bowel
    - domestic violence.

Examination reveals spontaneous rupture of the membranes at 26 weeks – uterus relaxed, cephalic presentation.

Marks will be awarded for:

- discussing appropriate management:
    - blood investigations
    - swabs
    - ultrasound
    - conservative management – antibiotics
    - steroids
- overall sympathetic approach.

Khaled M Khaled, Roopa Nair and Barry Whitlow

Station 42

You are asked to see 42-year-old Mrs Weaver in the gynaecology clinic. The GP has sent you a letter stating that she suffers from heavy periods. You are to take a history and discuss management options with her. Examination findings will be provided.

Marks will be awarded for:

- appropriate introduction, eye contact and nonmedical language
- obtaining relevant history:
  - overweight
  - history of intermenstrual/postcoital bleeding
  - previous surgeries
  - past history of DVT
  - previous Mirena use
  - last smear
  - social and family history.

Examination findings are normal.

Marks will be awarded for:

- discussing appropriate investigations:
  - full blood count
  - ultrasound scan
  - Pipelle endometrial sampling
  - thyroid and hormone tests not indicated
  - hysteroscopy
- discussing treatment options
  - endometrial ablation
  - hysterectomy.

Patient chooses hysterectomy.

Marks will be awarded for:

- discussing oophorectomy
- asking about total versus subtotal – to discuss.

Station 43

You are given an instrument (forceps) used in routine obstetric practice. Discuss the instrument with the examiner.

Marks will be awarded for:

- correctly describing the various features of forceps
- indications (must be described to RCOG standards)
- contraindications (must be described to RCOG standards)
- prerequisites for forceps application (ask yourself whether you are the right operator, is the woman the right patient and whether the instrument is appropriate)
- describe application and delivery (depending upon type of forceps given)
- complications:
  - maternal
  - fetal
- cord gases
- third stage
- rectal and vaginal examinations
- documentation.

Station 44

You are given an instrument (hysteroscope) used in routine gynaecological practice. Discuss the instrument with the examiner.

Marks will be awarded for:

- assembling hysteroscope correctly
- explaining procedure correctly
- knowledge of various distension media – saline, CO_2, glycine
- indications (these must be well understood):
  - diagnostic
  - therapeutic
- risks of hysteroscopy:
  - fluid overload
  - uterine perforation
- difficulties encountered during procedure:
  - false passage
  - blood

Q. What would you do if perforation is suspected during hysteroscopy?

Answer:

- Senior help
- Observation of vital signs
- Laparoscopy to rule out bowel injury and bleeding
- Antibiotics
- Debriefing.

Khaled M Khaled, Roopa Nair and Barry Whitlow

Station 45

You are given an instrument (laparoscope) used in routine gynaecological practice. Discuss the instrument with the examiner.

Marks will be awarded for:

- assembling laparoscope correctly
- explaining insertion with Veress needle and creation of pneumoperitoneum
- explaining insertion of trocar
- indications (these must be well understood):
  - diagnostic
  - therapeutic
- risks of laparoscopy:
  - bowel injury
  - major vessel injury
- difficulties encountered during insertion:
  - adhesions
  - blood
- alternative entry sites – Palmer's point

Q. What would you do in the case of accidental vessel injury during laparoscopy?

Answer:

- Do not move Veress needle
- Bloods – crossmatch
- Laparotomy
- Senior help
- Debriefing.

Station 46

You are asked to see Mrs Jones, a 30-year-old woman who is 38 weeks into her second pregnancy. She had an elective caesarean in her first pregnancy for breech presentation. The baby is now of average size with head 2/5ths palpable.

Discuss her further management.

Marks will be awarded for:

- appropriate introduction
- avoiding medical jargon
- discussing vaginal birth after caesarean:
  - ◆ success rate 75–80%
  - ◆ benefits of vaginal delivery
  - ◆ risks of vaginal delivery including scar rupture 0.2–0.8%
- discussing risks and benefits of lower segment caesarean section
- role of induction
- balanced discussion
- allowing patient to decide.

Station 47

Mrs Hobbs, a 28-year-old primigravida, has been referred to you in antenatal clinic. She is 36 weeks pregnant and ultrasound has confirmed breech presentation.

Advise her on the further management.

Marks will be awarded for:

- appropriate introduction
- avoiding medical jargon
- explaining breech presentation
- confirming placental position and liquor on ultrasound
- possibility of spontaneous version
- explaining external cephalic version – procedure, success and risks
- options of vaginal breech delivery and caesarean section
- results of Term Breech Trial
- risks and benefits of lower segment caesarean section and vaginal breech delivery
- balanced discussion.

Station 48

A 49-year-old woman, who underwent transabdominal hysterectomy and bilateral salpingo-oophorectomy for heavy periods, wishes to discuss hormone replacement therapy.

Marks will be awarded for:

- appropriate language, avoiding medical jargon
- vasomotor symptoms
- osteoporosis
- risk of:
  - breast cancer
  - coronary heart disease
  - stroke
  - thromboembolism
- current recommendations and studies – brief outline
- allowing patient to decide on risk/benefit ratio for her
- offering alternatives, e.g. selective estrogen receptor modulators (SERMs), venlafaxine, phytoestrogens.

Khaled M Khaled, Roopa Nair and Barry Whitlow

Station 49

You are the consultant in clinic. You are seeing Miss Dixon, a 19-year-old student, who is complaining of amenorrhoea and hirsutism. She is obese with a body mass index of 35. She has had various hormone investigations and a scan that is suggestive of polycystic ovaries.

You are seeing her to explain the diagnosis and offer her a management plan.

Marks will be awarded for:

- sensitive and sympathetic approach
- avoiding medical jargon while explaining diagnosis
- inviting questions and checking whether the patient understands
- discussing patient's priorities
- discussing implications of polycystic ovaries
- offering lifestyle advice and discussing weight loss sensitively
- treatment for for hirsutism: cosmetic measures, medical management
- implications for future fertility (discuss options only if patient asks)
- offering follow-up visit
- sensitive discussion of health issues such as diabetes and cardiovascular risks (may be discussed at follow-up visits).

Station 50

You are the registrar in clinic and are seeing Mrs Thrower, a 29-year-old nulliparous woman, who has suffered from amenorrhoea for 1 year. She wants to conceive and therefore saw her GP, who conducted some blood tests. All her test results, including hormone assays, are normal except the following:

LH   52 iu/l
FSH   96 iu/l

Marks will be awarded for:

- sensitive and sympathetic approach
- avoiding medical jargon, inviting questions, checking whether patient understands
- discussing patient's priorities
- premature ovarian failure: discussing implications, effects on bone and cardiovascular system (remember the effects) with relevant advice
- hormone replacement therapy
- karyotyping and further investigations
- counselling
- fertility issues – ovum donation and IVF
- lifestyle advice about osteoporosis, cardiovascular risk
- offering follow-up visit.

Khaled M Khaled, Roopa Nair and Barry Whitlow

Station 51

Mrs Cowley attends the family planning clinic for her Depo Provera® injection. She has been using Depo Provera as her chosen method of contraception for the past 4 years and has been amenorrhoeic since then.

She is a 47-year-old secretary who smokes 30 cigarettes a day and consumes 23 units of alcohol per week. She has no children but had a termination of pregnancy in her teens. Recent cervical smear tests have been normal but she had a cone biopsy in her 20s. She has been in a new relationship for the past 9 months. She is slim but has a strong family history of heart disease; her father died of a myocardial infarction at 44 years of age.

Her mother died of a pulmonary embolus following a fractured neck of femur at 57 years of age. Mrs Cowley suffers from asthma, which is controlled by a combination of Salbutamol and steroid inhalers. About two to three times a year she needs oral steroids. She has tried to stop smoking but has been unable to do so. In the past, she has suffered with heavy, painful menses. She wants to continue with Depo Provera. Neither she nor her partner like using barrier methods.

Q. What issues would you want to discuss with Mrs C?

Answer:

- Long-term use of Depo Provera – effects on bone density.
- Risk factors for osteoporosis – smoking, alcohol, family history, steroids, slim, early menopause.
- Menopause – is she menopausal? Relevance of blood tests (FSH), fertility in older women, need for effective contraception.
- Relevance of family history – father and myocardial infarction age 44 years; mother and pulmonary embolism (unlikely she will need clotting screen but may need to be considered).
- Menstrual history; suitability for different contraception, e.g. combined oral contraceptives, progestogen-only pill, Implanon, intrauterine device, levonorgestrel-releasing intrauterine system.
- Possible need for sexually transmitted disease screening – new relationship; pre-IUD/LNG-IUS.

- LNG-IUS – benefits: effect on menstruation (previous menorrhagia, early spotting and possible amenorrhoea after insertion, menopausal symptoms and ability to check FSH levels), contraception, endometrial protection (if requires HRT).
- LNG-IUS – insertion procedure: possibly more difficult as only one termination of pregnancy and previous cone biopsy.

Station 52

Ms Howard is a 19-year-old university student. She had a termination of pregnancy at the age of 17 years. She smokes five cigarettes a day and is taking low-dose tetracycline for acne. She has no significant medical history, is normotensive and has a body mass index of 25. She has been with her partner for 6 months and has been using Dianette for 4 months.

She attends the family planning clinic on Monday morning for further advice and gives the following history:

She had forgotten to take pill 3 from her packet of pills. She had intercourse the previous night and attended her GP the following day. He prescribed Levonelle 1500 and advised her to double the dose as she was taking antibiotics, to stop the Dianette and restart with her next period.

She took the 'double dose' and used condoms but 3 days later, the condom split.

She attended the walk-in centre the following day (Saturday) requesting emergency contraception again. She was advised that it could not be taken more than once in a cycle and that she should attend the family planning clinic on Monday morning to discuss insertion of an intrauterine device.

How would you have managed the client if you had been:

● the GP at the first visit?
● the health professional at the walk-in centre?
● the family planning doctor at the third visit?

Are there any other issues that you would wish to raise?

Answer:

● Current recommendations (World Health Organization, Faculty of Family Planning and Reproductive Health Care of the RCOG, fpa) for missed combined pills are that it is acceptable to miss one 20-microgram pill or two 30-microgram pills at any time in the cycle.

- These new recommendations state that:
  - pill-taking should continue as usual
  - it is not necessary to use other precautions in this instance
  - emergency contraception is not necessary.
- Additional precautions are now only advised if two 20-microgram or three 30-microgram pills are missed. Some professionals dispute this but even the 'old' ruling stated that emergency contraception was only necessary if two or more pills of numbers one to seven were missed and intercourse had taken place.
- Following current recommendations, the advice from the GP should have been that she did not need emergency contraception. She should have been advised to continue pill-taking as usual and did not need to use condoms for the next 7 days. There would also have been no need to increase the dose of Levonelle, as the efficacy of progestogen-only contraceptives is not affected by antibiotics.
- The efficacy of oestrogen-containing contraceptives can be affected by non-enzyme-inducing antibiotics but the large bowel flora will re-establish themselves in about 2 weeks so precautions are only advised if a woman starts or changes a long-term antibiotic when already on the combined oral contraceptive pill (for 3 weeks) or if she has been taking the antibiotics for less than 3 weeks when she commences her first packet.
- Emergency contraception is only licensed to be given once in a cycle but it is accepted practice (WHO, FFPRHC) that it can be prescribed more than once in the same cycle. The first act of unprotected sexual intercourse took place on day nine from the start of the pill-free interval; the second act took place on day 13/14 from the start of the pill-free interval. One of the actions of emergency contraception is to inhibit or delay ovulation so she is possibly more likely to be at risk of an unplanned pregnancy at this point in the cycle.
- When she attended the family planning clinic on Monday morning, she was still within the 72 hours since unprotected sexual intercourse and could have been offered emergency hormonal contraception. However, Levonelle is most effective if given as soon as possible after unprotected sexual intercourse and a copper-IUD is more effective at any time. A copper-IUD can be fitted up to day 19 of a 28-day cycle regardless of the number of times unprotected sexual intercourse has taken place.

Station 53

You are presented with a selection of methods of contraception and asked the following questions:

- Can you name any of these female methods of contraception?
- What is their contraceptive efficacy?
- In what range of sizes are the different types available?
- Do women need to have a fitting to assess the correct size?
- If so, when can this be done after:
  - pregnancy?
  - termination?
- When/how often should the fitting be rechecked?
- Should they all/always be used with spermicides?
- How long should they be left in place before being removed?
- What about women with a latex sensitivity?
- Can they be damaged by the use of oil-based lubricants? Name some oil-based lubricants.
- What diaphragm/caps are most suitable for a woman with a posteriorly positioned cervix?
- Which diaphragms/caps are most suitable for a woman with a lax vagina?
- What spermicidal agent is contained in the creams/gels/pessaries? Are there any health issues connected with the use of spermicides?

Answer:

- Identification: flat-spring diaphragm; arcing diaphragm; Dumas (vault) cap; Vimule; cervical (Prentif) cap; Femcap; Femidom.
- Contraceptive efficacy: 4–20/100 women years (higher efficacy applies to older women and more experienced users (spermicides alone are highly ineffective and not recommended).
- Sizes:
  - flat-spring and arcing diaphragms: nine sizes from 55 mm to 95 mm
  - Dumas: five sizes from 50 mm to 75 mm
  - Vimule: three sizes of 42 mm, 48 mm and 54 mm
  - cervical cap: four sizes of 22 mm, 25 mm, 28 mm and 31 mm

- ◆ Femcap: three sizes of 22 mm, 26 mm and 30 mm
- ◆ Femidom: one size only.
- Women need fitting for all types of cap/diaphragm except Femcap. Can be done 6 weeks after delivery or immediately after termination.
- After 1–2 weeks to check the fitting and then check annually but a recheck should be advised after pregnancy, vaginal surgery or with a weight gain or loss of 4 kg.
- Additional spermicide is recommended with all types except Femidom.
- They can be inserted any time before intercourse but if this is longer than 2 hours, additional spermicide must be used. It should be left in position for at least 6 hours after the last intercourse but additional spermicide must be added if intercourse takes place again during that time.
- Femcap is a silicon cap and Femidom is made from polyurethane – these are the only barrier methods designed for women that are latex free.
- Potentially, they can be damaged by the use of oil-based lubricants; it is recommended that oil-based lubricants are avoided. This does not apply to Femcap or Femidom. Oil-based lubricants include: vaseline, baby oil, petroleum jelly, skin and suntan lotions, oestrogen creams (Premarin, Orthodienoestrol), antifungal preparations (not Canesten).
- For a woman with a posteriorly positioned cervix: arcing diaphragms.
- For a woman with a lax vagina: cervical cap.
- Spermicidal agent: nonoxynol-9. Studies have highlighted the concern that frequent use of N-9 may damage the vaginal mucosa and increase the chance of HIV transmission.

Index

Khaled M Khaled, Roopa Nair and Barry Whitlow